Nursing

Mnemonics

117 TIPS, TRICKS, AND MEMORY CUES TO HELP YOU KICK-ASS IN NURSING SCHOOL

Chris Mulder, CRNA, MSN

Contents

About the Author

My name is Chris Mulder, a full-time nurse anesthetist at a level 1 trauma center in Central Florida. Long before becoming a CRNA, I worked in a tiny cubicle all day in a position that rendered my English degree useless. That only lasted a couple of years before I realized something had to change before I lost my mind. Much to my wife's dismay, I decided to go back to school to get my nursing degree. It wasn't easy, but I made it through. After graduation, I worked as a registered nurse in the medical ICU in a large hospital in Lakeland, FL. A few years later, I applied for Nurse Anesthesia School, and the rest is history!

As I've gone through my years of training and working as a nurse, I've come to realize a few things. The information I was getting in the classroom was difficult to retain and rarely translated to real-world practice. I also found that most nurses took themselves too seriously and were often condescending. That's why I try to keep things a little more light-hearted without all the arrogance.

I know what you're going through. I remember the constant struggle and the sleepless nights. I know the butterflies in the stomach before clinicals and the sinking feeling right before submitting an exam. Stick with me and we'll get through this together. I

might be a nurse anesthetist, but I am a NURSE
before anything else.

Introduction

Mnemonics can be a great tool to help your brain trigger specific information that you need to know quickly. This tactic can be used for exams, during questioning by instructors, or in your everyday clinical practice. It should be noted that memory tricks like these should not be thought of as a replacement for knowledge of the subject. You first need to understand the core concepts before the mnemonics will be able to help.

The good news is that once you have a grasp on the material you are trying to learn, mnemonics can make your life much easier. This is especially true in the world of nursing. There are thousands of diagnoses, labs, medications, symptoms, and treatments. Even after you learn something new, it is easy to get things mixed up.

For example, does your patient have dysphagia or aphasia or dysphasia or aphagia? What!? I feel your pain. Don't worry, this is covered later, along with tons of other difficult-to-remember nursing topics.

The idea here isn't to read this entire book to try to remember every single mnemonic. You'll drive yourself crazy that way. Rather, it is meant to be used as a guide as you progress through nursing school and even as you begin your career as a nurse.

When you start to cover a specific topic in school, come back to this book and see if there is a mnemonic for it. If you've graduated and there is something you just can't seem to remember, see if we have something that will help. This way, you will be learning as you go, and will be less likely to get the mnemonics mixed up.

Also, keep in mind that mnemonics will never have all of the possible information for a specific topic. Only the most important things are covered, and sometimes items are left out for the sake of the mnemonic. It would be impossible to condense a 50-page chapter on electrolytes into a few words.

Some of these mnemonic devices are commonly known and I have used them myself many times. However, the majority of them are original creations by yours truly. Some of them may sound strange and funny. But this is a good thing! Those are the ones you are more likely to remember.

If something in this book just doesn't seem to be working for you, try to come up with your own mnemonic for that subject. It's not hard. Just try putting letters together to make up words or sentences that you can draw from when the time comes.

If you have any questions about anything in this book, please feel free to email me at contact@kickassnursing.com. Visit us on our web site at www.kickassnursing.com and check out the blog and our other books to help you get through nursing school. Enjoy the mnemonics!

FLUIDS AND ELECTROLYTES

Hypercalcemia – Symptoms

MANIAC

Muscle weakness
Abdominal pain
Nausea/vomiting
Increased urine/thirst
Aching bones
Confusion

Alternative...

BONES, GROANS, STONES, and MOANS

BONES (Painful Bones)
GROANS (Abdominal Pain)
STONES (Kidney Stones)
MOANS (Psychiatric – Confusion, Depression)

Calcium is an important electrolyte, affecting many body systems. Its effects are very apparent in the musculoskeletal system, as it is prevalent in this area. Hypercalcemia can cause muscle weakness and aching bones. Build-up in the urinary system can cause kidney stones, abdominal pain, and nausea. It also acts in the neurological system, which is why your patient might be confused. Hypercalcemia can also cause major issues in the cardiac tissue, which can manifest as arrhythmias and ekg changes.

Hypercalcemia – Treatment

<u>CHEFS</u>

<u>C</u>alcitonin

<u>H</u>ydration/fluids

<u>E</u>ase symptoms

<u>F</u>orced Diuresis

<u>S</u>odium Intake, <u>S</u>urgery

To treat hypercalcemia, you must correct the underlying problem and replace it as necessary. Calcitonin is a hormone in the body that reduces calcium levels. These patients are usually dehydrated, so fluids are a priority. Increasing the salt intake will cause the body to get rid of calcium in the urine. Once the patient is adequately hydrated, loop diuretics can be helpful in this regard. Avoid thiazide diuretics as they can increase calcium even more. Surgery may be needed if the problem is the parathyroid gland.

Hypocalcemia – Symptoms

SPASTICS

Spasms (muscle spasms, laryngospasms)

Paresthesias

Arrhythmias

Stridor

Trousseau sign

Irritability

Chvostek sign

Seizures

Hypocalcemia can cause spasms if the muscles don't have enough to work with. It can also cause seizures, as calcium is important for the neurological system. Calcium is also vital for the heart to function, so you may see arrhythmias. Low calcium can cause the larynx to spasm, which may present as stridor. Chvostek Sign can be checked by tapping on the facial nerve on the cheek. A positive sign would be contractions in that area. Trousseau Sign is when you see carpal spasm during blood pressure cuff inflation.

Hyperkalemia - Symptoms

<u>WHINERS</u>

<u>W</u>eak muscles/cramps

<u>H</u>ypotension

<u>I</u>rritability

<u>N</u>ausea/vomiting/diarrhea

<u>E</u>kg Changes

<u>R</u>espiratory distress

<u>S</u>low heart rate (bradycardia)

Hyperkalemia can be caused by many things, but is most commonly due to renal insufficiency or failure. It is one of the most important electrolytes in the body, affecting many systems. It plays a major role in the proper functioning of the muscles in the body, which is why your patient might get muscle cramps. In an attempt to get rid of the excess, you may see vomiting and diarrhea. Ekg changes are common, as potassium has a major effect on the heart. Extreme hyperkalemia can cause cardiac arrest, which is why it is used in lethal injection.

Hyperkalemia – EKG Changes

<u>WASP</u>

Widened QRS

Arrhythmias

ST Depression

Peaked T wave

One of the most important effects of hyperkalemia is evident in the heart and is often displayed as ekg changes. The earliest manifestation is usually peaked t waves. At very high levels, you will also see arrhythmias. It might start out with simple PACs and PVCs, but can quickly progress to ventricular fibrillation and asystole if left untreated.

Hyperkalemia – Treatment

C A BIG K+ Drop

Calcium

Albuterol

Bicarbonate/**B**eta agonists
Insulin
Glucose

Kayexelate

Dialysis/**D**iet/**D**iuretics/**D**50

While calcium won't directly lower the potassium, it allows for stabilization of the heart muscle. Beta-2 agonists (albuterol), Insulin, and Bicarbonate help by driving potassium back into the cell. This decreases the overall extracellular potassium, which is the form that can cause effects on the body. Glucose is given with insulin simply to prevent hypoglycemia. Kayexelate binds with potassium in the intestine and gets excreted in the feces. You can also restrict the potassium in the diet, or you can give diuretics to get rid of it through the urine. Lastly, dialysis is usually needed, especially for renal failure patients. Though the other treatments will help to decrease it temporarily, the underlying problem must be dealt with.

Hypokalemia – Symptoms

WILDCATS

Weakness

Ileus/**I**ntestinal motility decreased

Lethargy

Diarrhea/nausea/vomiting

Confusion

Arrhythmias/**A**lkalosis

Thready pulse

Shallow respirations

Just as too much potassium can cause problems, too little potassium can do the same thing. Patients often have little or no symptoms at first. If it gets too low, they may start to have generalized weakness and confusion, and possibly some muscle cramping. If it gets very low, you will begin to see ekg changes such as prolonged QT, but can quickly progress to ventricular tachycardia and ventricular fibrillation. As the muscles get weaker, patients may have difficulty breathing.

Hypokalemia – Treatment

DIP

Diet
IV Replacement
Potassium Sparing Diuretics/**P**O Replacement

The treatment for hypokalemia is fairly simple. You must first figure out what's causing the potassium to drop, and then you must replace it. The easiest way to replace it is by giving a regular dose by mouth. If somewhat rapid correction is needed, or if the patient is NPO, then IV replacement can be utilized. Once stabilized, look for things in the diet that are high in potassium and encourage them. If the patient is on a diuretic, consider switching to one that is potassium-sparing. Check the potassium on a regular basis to make sure the patient doesn't become hyperkalemic.

Hypermagnesemia – Symptoms

WARMTH

Weakness

Arrhythmias

Respiratory failure

Muscle fatigue

Tired

Hypotension

Magnesium is another important electrolyte in the body, though is usually not considered a priority. It is not part of the BMP, so must be ordered separately along with the phosphate. It is important for muscles, which is why you may see muscle weakness and general fatigue. It also plays a big role in cardiac function. These patients may have arrhythmias and low blood pressure.

Hypomagnesemia – Symptoms

FLATTEN

Fasciculations

Lethargy

Anorexia

Tetany

Tremor

Exhaustion

Nausea

Since magnesium is important for muscles, you may see fasciculations, tremor, and tetany when it's low. Lethargy, nausea, loss of appetite, and exhaustion. A very low magnesium level may cause an arrhythmia called Torsades de Pointes, which means "twisting of the points." If you see something like this on the ekg, think about hypomagnesemia.

Hypernatremia – Symptoms

FAINTED

Fever, Flushed skin

Anxiety, confusion

Increased Blood Pressure (hypertension)

Nausea

Thirst

Edema

Decreased urine output

Alternative...

FRIED

Fever, Flushed skin

Restless, anxious, confused

Increased blood pressure (hypertension)

Edema

Dry Mouth, thirst

A high sodium level can have effects on many body systems, with the major concern being neurological. These patients can often get confused, have seizures, and even go into a coma. However, these happen usually when the sodium is very high. Initial symptoms include thirst and dry mouth. You may see nausea and vomiting, as well as hypertension and low urine output. The sodium is usually high because the patient is dehydrated, but can be due to other reasons also.

Hyponatremia – Symptoms

CHEWS

Confusion, **C**oma, muscle **C**ramps

Headache

Emesis (nausea/vomiting)

Weakness

Seizures

Hyponatremia can be even more of a concern than hypernatremia. Again, you may see nausea and vomiting. These patients can also get bad headaches, as well as seizures and muscle cramps. At very low levels, the patient may go into a coma. It's important to bring the sodium level back up slowly, as quick replacement can cause major neurological damage.

Hypovolemic Shock – Symptoms

TIPTOE

Tachycardia

Increased SVR

Poor skin turgor

Thirst

Oliguria (decreased urine)

Extreme weakness

Hypovolemic Shock happens when there is not enough volume, fluid or blood, circulating throughout the body. Common symptoms include tachycardia, increased systemic vascular resistance, poor skin turgor, thirst, decreased urine output, and extreme weakness. If you know the signs of dehydration, then you know the signs for hypovolemic shock. Just imagine it as a much more severe case.

CARDIO-VASCULAR SYSTEM

Adrenergic Receptors

Beta-1 affects the Heart (**1 Heart**)

Beta-2 affects the Lungs (**2 Lungs**)

Beta-1 and beta-2 are adrenergic receptors. There is also an alpha-1, alpha-2, and beta-3. Learn those also, but the two most common you'll see in nursing school will likely be beta-1 and beta-2. Beta-1 receptors primarily affect the heart. For example, beta-1 agonists help to increase cardiac output and heart rate. Beta-2 receptors primarily affect the lungs. For example, beta-2 agonists help to relax the smooth muscle in the lungs, causing bronchial dilation. These are commonly used in the treatment of asthma.

Cardiac Conduction – Electrical Pathway

On **Sa**turdays, I **Av**oid **B**ee **H**ives with **B**umble **B**ees in the **P**ark **F**orest

SA Node – **AV** Node – **B**undle of **H**IS – **B**undle **B**ranches (right and left) – **P**urkinje's **F**ibers

When I was in school, I had a heck of a time remembering two things: the blood flow through the heart and the conduction pathway through the heart. This mnemonic isn't ideal, but it helped me recall it in a pinch. The first signal comes from the sinoatrial (SA) node and proceeds to the atrioventricular (AV) node. From here, the signal goes to the Bundle of HIS and then to the right and left bundle branches. Finally, the electrical current gets to the Purkinje's Fibers.

Cardiac Tamponade – Symptoms

"Beck's Triad" in **3D**

Distant heart sounds
Decreased arterial BP
Distended jugular veins

Alternative...

Have **M**ore **J**uice

Hypotension
Muffled heart sounds
JVD (Jugular vein distention)

Cardiac tamponade is when there is so much f fluid around the heart that it causes compression, decreasing the strength at which the heart can work. Common signs and symptoms include distant heart sounds, hypotension, and distended jugular veins. Together, these encompass what's referred to as Beck's Triad. Follow one or both of these mnemonics to help you remember.

Cardiogenic Shock – Source

RIP

Rhythm
Ischemia
Pump

Cardiogenic shock happens when there isn't enough blood flow in the body due to heart failure. This could be because of the heart rhythm, ischemia, and pump problems. If the heart is in a rhythm that can't maintain perfusion, it could lead to cardiogenic shock (supraventricular tachycardia, atrial fibrillation, etc). If there is a lack of blood flow getting to the heart, such as in myocardial ischemia, it could also cause this problem. The heart muscle can get weaker, making it less effective. This is the most common reason. The last cause of cardiogenic shock in this mnemonic, "pump," is when the heart isn't pumping properly because of a mechanical issue like endocarditis, valve disorders, or cardiomyopathies.

Cardiogenic Shock – Treatment

HABIT

Hydrate
Anti-arrhythmics
Balloon pump (intra-aortic)
Inotropes
Treat symptoms

Cardiogenic shock happens when there isn't enough blood flow in the body due to heart failure. Treatment goals will be to increase the heart's strength and ability to pump. Depending on the underlying problem, the patient will need to be given fluids, anti-arrhythmics, inotropes, and even an intra-aortic balloon pump if necessary. As with anything else, treat the symptoms as they arise.

Circulation Through the Heart

I **S**aw the **RAT** **R**ead **V**ampire **P**oems, while his **PAL** **P**layed **V**iolin, **L**ooking **A**t **M**y **L**unch **V**ery **AA**nxiously

IVC + **S**VC > **R**ight **A**trium > **T**ricuspid Valve > **R**ight **V**entricle > **P**ulmonary valve > **P**ulmonary **A**rteries > **L**ungs > **P**ulmonary **V**eins > **L**eft **A**trium > **M**itral valve > **L**eft **V**entricle > **A**ortic Valve > **A**orta

Heart Valves in Order

Toilet **P**aper **M**y **A**ss

Tricuspid

Pulmonary

Mitral

Aortic

Circulation through the heart is tricky to learn. I know that the mnemonic on the top is very difficult and may not help at all. This is a topic that may just require straight memorization. But I thought I'd give it a shot anyway. The bottom mnemonic for the heart valves may be a little more helpful.

CHF (Congestive Heart Failure) – Treatment

UNLOAD FAST

Upright position
Nitrates
Lasix
Oxygen
ACE Inhibitors
Digoxin

Fluid restriction
Afterload reduction
Sodium restriction
Tests (digoxin level, ABGs, BNP)

For a patient with CHF, you are going to want to "UNLOAD" the extra fluid "FAST." Keep these patients in the upright position to help facilitate breathing and make them more comfortable. Nitrates may be ordered to help decrease demand on the heart. They may need oxygen to help ventilation, but also to get more oxygen to the heart. To reduce fluid, diuretics such as Lasix can be given. These patients should also be put on fluid restrictions and a low sodium diet. Water follows sodium, so the more salt in their diet, the more water will hang around. ACE inhibitors can be used to treat hypertension, something common in this patient population. Digoxin can help to improve the strength of each heart contraction and aid in circulation. These patients should have regular labs done, such as ABGs and BNP levels. If they are on digoxin, they will need to have digoxin levels checked.

EKG Basics

PAC the things from **QVC TV R**apidly

P wave: **A**trial **C**ontraction (depolarization)
QRS: **V**entricular **C**ontraction (depolarization)
T wave: **V**entricular **R**epolarization

This one is tough, but so many people have a hard time remembering exactly what they're looking at when they look at an ekg, some mnemonic had to be considered. Good luck—I hope you can think of a better one. The way I remember it is by using the phrase "Pack the things from QVC TV Rapidly." In case you weren't aware, QVC is a program on TV where you can call in or go online to buy things while they are on sale for a short period of time. So, come with me on this silly mnemonic journey.

After you buy them, you want to **PAC**k them up. The **P** wave on an ekg represents depolarization, or **A**trial **C**ontraction.

You bought the things from **QVC**. The **Q**RS complex on an ekg represents a continuing part of depolarization, or **V**entricular **C**ontraction.

You didn't just buy the things from QVC—you bought them on **TV R**apidly. The **T** wave on an ekg represents **V**entricular **R**epolarization.

EKG Lead Placement

For a standard 5 lead ekg, follow these simple rules to remember where they go on the chest.

1. Smoke over Fire (<u>Black over Red</u>)

2. <u>White</u> on Right

3. <u>Green</u>: Gallbladder

4. <u>Brown</u> "Around" the Sternum

As easy as this sounds, a basic 5-lead ekg lead placement still gets misplaced by even the most seasoned nurses. But it's so simple if you can remember this mnemonic. Start with the left side: smoke over fire. Think of the black lead as the smoke and place it in the upper left half of the body (usually near the left shoulder/chest). The red lead (fire) should then be placed under the black lead on the lower half of the body (typically on the lower left abdomen or ribcage). Once you have these two, move on to the next part of the mnemonic.

The white lead placement should be easy to remember because it rhymes with right, which is where it needs to be. This is typically placed opposite of the black lead and is usually around the right shoulder/chest area. The green lead is the only lead that starts with 'G', just like the word, 'gallbladder,' This lead should be on the lower right side of the body and is usually placed in the general area of the gallbladder (in the lower right abdomen or ribcage). Finally, the brown lead should be placed 'around' the sternum (brown: around). For basic 5 lead in V1 position, this is just to the right of mid-sternum.

Heart Blocks

Popular poem to help remember the different types of heart block

1st Degree: If R is far from P, we call that a 1st degree

2nd Degree, Type 1 (Wenkebach): Longer, longer, longer, drop. Now we have a Wenkebach

2nd Degree, Type 2 (Mobitz II): If some P's just can't get through, now we have a Mobitz II

3rd Degree (Complete Heart Block): If the P's and Q's cannot agree, now we have a 3rd degree

1st degree heart block is characterized by a P-R interval greater than 0.2 seconds. It looks like a typical sinus rhythm, but the p wave is farther from the r wave than normal.

2nd degree, type 1 heart block is also known as a Wenkebach. You may see or hear either term. In this type of block, the p wave goes further away from the r wave with each beat. Eventually, a beat is skipped and the cycle starts over.

2nd degree, type II heart block is also known as a Mobitz II. In this type of block, the rhythm appears normal until a complex suddenly gets dropped without warning. The P-R interval is constant and it just looks like a beat gets skipped.

3rd degree heart block, also known as complete heart block, is where the P waves and the QRS complex don't communicate with each other at all. There is no rhyme or reason where a P wave or a QRS will show up.

Heart Failure – Left Sided

POACHED

Pulmonary congestion
Orthopnea
Adventitious breath sounds
Cough
Hemoptysis
Extreme weakness
Dyspnea

Alternative...

SCORED

Sleepy (fatigue)
Cyanosis/**C**onfusion
Orthopnea
Rales/**R**estlessness
Extreme weakness
Dyspnea

Left sided heart failure happens when the left ventricle isn't pumping effectively enough. Since it's not getting blood out of the heart in sufficient volumes, fluid builds up into the lungs, causing pulmonary edema. These patients will have difficulty breathing and will be very weak. They might have a cough and sometimes you see hemoptysis (pink frothy sputum is a hallmark symptom). The lungs will sound wet in the form of rales or crackles.

Heart Failure – Right Sided

BOUNCED

Bloating

Oliguria

Unable to eat

Nausea

Cyanosis/**C**ool legs

Edema

Distended neck veins (JVD)

Alternative...

WARHEAD

Weight gain (because of retained fluid)

Anorexia

Reduced urine output

Hepatomegaly

Edema

Ascites

Distended neck veins (JVD)

Right sided heart failure usually happens when fluid in the lungs causes the right ventricle to work harder and eventually pump less effectively. Although some other factors could be in play, it is usually left-sided heart failure that causes it. It's like a vicious cycle. The left ventricle can't clear fluid from the lungs and the right ventricle has a difficult time pumping against that extra fluid. When the right ventricle fails, fluid will start to back up to the rest of the body. Common symptoms include generalized edema, ascites, jugular venous distention, enlarged liver, decreased urine output, loss of appetite, nausea, and weight gain (due to the retained fluid).

Heart Sounds

Lub Dub
S1 (Lub) + S2(Dub)

Which Valves Close During S1 and S2?

Some **1 Tr**icked **M**e
S1: **Tr**icuspid and **M**itral valves

2 Apple **P**ies
S**2**: **A**ortic and **P**ulmonary valves

During S1, the tricuspid and mitral valves close. The mitral valve closure typically happens slightly before the tricuspid valve closure. This is the beginning of ventricular contraction (systole). During S2 is when the aortic and pulmonic valves close. Normally, the aortic valve closes slightly before the pulmonic valve. This signifies the end of ventricular systole and the start of ventricular diastole.

Sometimes, an S3 sound can be heard. In a young, healthy patient and sometimes in pregnancy, this can be benign. However, it may also indicate CHF if it happens later in life. S4 can also be heard in conditions such as hypertension, aortic stenosis, or cardiomyopathy.

Location for Heart Sounds

APE To Man

Aortic

Pulmonary

Erb's Point

Tricuspid

Mitral

Alternative...

All People Enjoy Time Magazine

Aortic

Pulmonary

Erb's Point

Tricuspid

Mitral

This mnemonic should help you remember where to hear the different heart sounds when listening with a stethoscope. You should be able to hear the aortic valve at the right 2nd intercostal space and the pulmonic valve at the left 2nd intercostal space. Erb's point can be heard by auscultating at the left 3rd intercostal space. It is here that the S1 and S2 hearts sounds can best be found. You can hear the tricuspid valve at the left lower sternal border, adjacent to the 4th intercostal space. Finally, the mitral valve should be auscultated at the left 5th intercostal space, just medial to the midclavicular line.

If you can remember APE To Man and you can remember to start listening at the right 2nd intercostal space, you should be good to go. From there, shift left, and then down one by one for the others.

Hypertension - Complications

The 5 C's

CAD (coronary artery disease)

CRF (chronic renal failure)

CHF (congestive heart failure)

CVA (cerebrovascular accident)

Cardiac Arrest

Also part of the DIURETIC mnemonic, the 5 C's represent some common complications of hypertension. Coronary artery disease, chronic renal failure, congestive heart failure, cerebrovascular accidents, and cardiac arrest are all very big concerns for the patient with chronically high blood pressure. These things should be monitored for closely, using available preventative measures, as well as treatments if necessary.

Hypertension – Management

DIURETIC

Daily weight
Intake and output
Urine production
Response of blood pressure
Electrolytes
Take pulses
Ischemic episodes
Complications (5 c's)

Patients with hypertension can have many complications, so many things will need to be monitored. A good way to remember those things is with the word, 'DIURETIC,' a drug class often used to treat hypertension. Patients with high blood pressure are sometimes overloaded with fluid, so it's important to remember to check their fluid intake and output, as well as their daily weight and urine production. If they are on a diuretic, electrolytes must be monitored, as many types of this drug can cause electrolyte disturbances. Don't forget to check their pulse. Tachycardia is common, but some medications can also cause an increase or decrease in heart rate. Once the patient is being treated with medications and other modalities, make sure you monitor their response to these treatments. If it's not working or working too much, then it will need to be adjusted accordingly.

Patients with high blood pressure are at a much higher risk for ischemic events, such as myocardial infarction, stroke, or pulmonary embolism. The 5 C's represent coronary artery disease, chronic renal failure, congestive heart failure, cardiac arrest, and cerebrovascular accident. These are all common complications of hypertension.

MI – Symptoms

CHEST WOUNDS

Chest pain
Heartburn
Exhaustion
Shortness of breath
Tachycardia

Weakness
Ominous feeling
Uneasiness
Nausea
Dizziness
Sweating

A heart attack (myocardial infarction) is not something to be taken lightly. If it doesn't kill you, then consider it a warning. The most obvious sign is chest pain that may radiate to the left arm and the back. Sometimes, it may present as stomach pain or heartburn. These patients are usually short of breath and are sweating. They may feel dizzy, nauseated, or may just have a general feeling of impending doom. If you spot a heart attack, treat it quickly to prevent lasting damage.

MI – Treatment

MOAN

Morphine

Oxygen

Aspirin

Nitrates

Alternative...

DBOOBS

Dilate (nitrates)

Beta Blocker

Oxygen

Opioids

Blood thinners

Surgery (cardiac cath, CABG)

Early treatment of a heart attack is vital to prevent further damage to the myocardium. Initial treatment includes nitroglycerin, oxygen, aspirin, and an opioid, such as morphine. Once the extent and location of the damage is confirmed, surgery may be needed, such as a CABG or a simple stent placement. These patients should be put on blood thinners to prevent future clot-related incidents.

Pacemaker Codes

PaSeR

Pa – Chamber **Pa**ced
Se – Chamber **Se**nsed
R – **R**esponse to sensing

First Letter – Chamber Paced
Second Letter – Chamber Sensed
Third Letter – Response to Sensing

Example: VVI = Ventricular Paced, Ventricular Sensed, Inhibited Mode

This mnemonic will help you remember what the pacemaker codes mean if you're in a hurry. The first letter represents the chamber of the heart that's being paced. The second letter represents the chamber of the heart that is being sensed. The third letter represents the pacemaker's response to sensing. Think about the word "pacer" with an S instead of a C. Then you have the Pa to represent the chamber Paced, the Se to represent the chamber Sensed, and the R to represent the pacemaker's Response to sensing.

ENDOCRINE SYSTEM

Addison's Disease - Causes

ADDISON

Autoimmune

Degenerative (amyloid)

Drugs (ketoconazole)

Infections

Secondary (Decreased ACTH, Hypopituitarism)

Others (Adrenal bleeding)

Neoplasia (Secondary carcinoma)

Addison's disease, also known as hypocortisolism, happens when there is not enough cortisol produced by the adrenal glands. It is an autoimmune disease that is degenerative in nature. Certain drugs, such as ketoconazole, inhibit cortisol synthesis and could help cause adrenal insufficiency. Infection, some carcinomas, decreased ACTH, and hypopituitarism can also cause Addison's disease. In rare instances, bleeding from the adrenal glands could lead to adrenal insufficiency.

Cushing Syndrome

CUSHING

<u>C</u>ollagen fiber weakness, <u>C</u>entral obesity

<u>U</u>rinary (Increased glucose and free cortisol)

<u>S</u>uppressed immunity

<u>H</u>ypertension, <u>H</u>yperlipidemia, <u>H</u>yperglycemia, <u>H</u>ypercortisolism

<u>I</u>ncreased corticosteroid use

<u>N</u>eoplasms

<u>G</u>lucose intolerance

Cushing Syndrome, also known as hypercortisolism, is a condition in which there is too much cortisol in the body. This can be caused by a problem in the body or by excessive and long-term use of corticosteroids. These patients often have very thin skin that is prone to bruising, due to collagen fiber weakness. They can also be obese, which may be due to fatty deposits (a buffalo hump appearance may be present in the back and shoulder area. There will be an increased amount of glucose and free cortisol in the urine. Their immune system will be depressed, and they usually have an intolerance to glucose. Hypertension and high cholesterol are also common findings.

DKA (Diabetic Ketoacidosis) – Treatment

*UCKING DKA

*Fluids
Urea (monitor it)
Creatinine (check it)
K+ (potassium – check and replace)
Insulin
NG tube
Glucose (give once levels begin to drop)

Diet (resume once DKA is resolved)
Keep track of Bicarb (give if needed to correct acidosis)
Anion gap (Get it less than 12)

The mnemonics with the curse words in them are usually the easiest to remember, and this one doesn't disappoint. Treatment for DKA is aimed at bringing the anion gap back below 12, so most of the measures here help to achieve that goal. Fluids are necessary to treat the obvious dehydration in these patients. Since they are so dehydrated, monitor their urea and creatinine to check the kidney function. Insulin will be needed to bring down the high glucose, but it should be dropped slowly and methodically. This insulin will often cause decreased potassium, so that will need to be monitored during treatment. Sodium Bicarbonate may be needed to help bring up the HCO3 in the blood. However, if treated properly, this should resolve eventually without it. A nasogastric tube might be necessary, particularly if the patient is comatose or very somnolent. Because of slow stomach digestion (gastroparesis), the NG tube will allow for suction of any excess contents to prevent regurgitation and aspiration into the lungs. Once the anion gap stabilizes, the glucose has a propensity to drop, especially if the insulin drip isn't stopped in time. Because of this, glucose may actually be needed at this time to prevent it from going too low.

Hyperglycemia – Symptoms

WHIPS

Weakness
Headaches
Increased thirst
Polyuria
Sight is blurry

This is a problem most often a concern for diabetic patients. Blood sugar that is out of control can cause headaches and weakness, as well as thirst and increased urine output (polyuria). Chronic hyperglycemia can lead to neuropathies, causing numbness and tingling in the extremities and even eye damage. If left untreated, it will cause problems with most organs in the body.

Hypoglycemia – Symptoms

TIRED CHAPS

Tachycardia
Irritability
Restlessness
Excessive hunger
Diaphoretic, **D**izzy

Confusion
Headache
Anxious
Pale
Syncope

Glucose is a major source of fuel for the neurological system. When it gets low, the primary symptoms reflect this. Patients will get pale and feel like they are going to faint. They feel weak and may be confused. They are dizzy, sweaty, and will usually have a high heart rate. If the glucose is not replaced quickly, they may eventually go into a coma. This could lead to permanent brain damage or even death.

Hyperthyroidism – Symptoms

THAWED

Tremors, **T**achycardia
Heat intolerance, **H**ypertension
Amenorrhea (menstrual changes)
Weight loss
Eyes bulging
Diarrhea

Hyperthyroidism may cause diarrhea and weight loss, along with tremors and tachycardia. These patients often have high blood pressure, weight loss, and bulging eyes. A hallmark symptom is an intolerance to heat. They often want the air conditioning turned down and the covers off. Think hyper = fast and hot.

Hypothyroidism – Symptoms

BEACHED WHALE

Brittle nails, **B**radycardia
Extreme fatigue
Apathy
Cold intolerance, **C**onstipation
Hair loss
Elevated cholesterol
Dry skin

Weight gain
Hairline receding
Anorexia
Lethargy
Edema (facial)

Patients with hypothyroidism will often have brittle nails, bradycardia, and are extremely tired and apathetic. They tend to gain weight, hold on to fluid (especially in their face), and have constipation. Sometimes they lose their hair, have dry and flaky skin, and a loss of appetite. A hallmark symptom is intolerance to cold, so these patients often like to wear warm clothes and may ask for blankets often. Think hypo = slow and cold.

Insulin

Rapid Acting:
Doesn't **LAG**

Lispro (Humalog)
Aspert (Novolog)
Glulisine (Apidra)

Sho**R**t Acting:
Remember the **R's**

Regular (Humulin **R**, Novolin **R**)

Intermediate Acting:
No **P**erson **H**ates **I**ce cream

NPH (Humulin N, Novolin N) – **I**ntermediate

Long Acting:
Life **D**etermines **G**lory

Long – **D**etemir (Levimir), **G**largine (Lantus)

Ultra-Long Acting:
U **L**ike **G**oofy **U**nderwear

Ultra-**L**ong – **G**largine **U**-500 (Toujee)

HEPATIC, RENAL, AND GI SYSTEMS

Appendicitis – Symptoms

FRY PANS

Fever
Rebound Tenderness (Mcburney's Point)
Young (peak incidence 10-12 years old)

Pain (right upper quadrant)
Anorexia
Nausea
Sudden relief may indicate rupture

Appendicitis is inflammation of the appendix. This is considered an emergency and usually needs to be treated surgically to remove the appendix. If not treated, it can rupture, allowing its contents to enter the abdominal cavity, which can eventually lead to sepsis. Common symptoms include fever, pain, loss of appetite, nausea and vomiting, and rebound tenderness (known as Mcburney's point—1/3 the distance from the anterior superior iliac spine to the umbilicus). These patients are typically young, as the peak incidence of appendicitis occurs from age 10-12. If these patients get sudden relief (without surgery), this can be indicative of rupture and should be treated immediately.

Bulimia vs Anorexia

Bulimia – **B**inges, then **B**lows chunks

Anorexia – **A**voids eating, **A**nxiety high

This one is going to be very basic for most of you, but I can remember getting these two definitions mixed up when I first started in nursing school. Use this mnemonic to remind you that bulimia means throwing up after eating, while anorexia means eating very little to nothing at times.

Cholecystitis – Risk Factors

5 F's

Fair skin (more common in Caucasians)
Fat (BMI >30)
Female
Fertile (1 or more children)
Forty (Age forty or older)

Cholecystitis is inflammation of the gallbladder. People at a higher risk fall into these five categories. Those with fair skin, who are obese, female, fertile, and at least 40 years old are at an increased risk of developing cholecystitis.

Cholecystitis – Symptoms

HAND FLIP

Hot (fever)
Anorexia
Nausea/vomiting
Distended abdomen

Feeling of fullness
Leukocytosis
Intolerance to fat
Pain (right upper quadrant)

Cholecystitis is inflammation of the gallbladder. Common symptoms in these patients include fever, loss of appetite, nausea and vomiting, distended abdomen, feeling of fullness, pain, intolerance to fat, and leukocytosis (elevated white blood count). The pain typically presents in the right upper quadrant of the abdomen.

Crohn's Disease – Symptoms

CHRISTMAS

Cobblestones (fissures and ulcers in the bowel that look like cobblestones)

High temperature

Reduced lumen

Intestinal fistulae

Skip lesions (patchy lesions that "skip" areas)

Transmural

Malabsorption

Abdominal pain

Submucosal fibrosis

Chron's disease is in inflammatory gastrointestinal condition that can cause severe abdominal pain. With these patients, you might see cobblestones, which are fissures and ulcers in the bowel. They may have a narrowed lumen in the intestines and intestinal fistulae can happen, in which fluid can leak into the abdominal cavity, possibly leading to sepsis. They may have skip lesions, which are patchy lesions that appear to skip in certain areas. Chron's disease is transmural, meaning it can affect the entire gastrointestinal tract, from the mouth to the anus. Malabsorption is common, preventing nutrients from being absorbed by the intestines. Finally, these patients may develop submucosal fibrosis, which is chronic fibrosis of the tissues in the mouth. This can eventually lead to jaw rigidity and the inability to open the mouth.

Cirrhosis Complications

I HAVE ASCITES

Increased bilirubin (causing jaundice)

Hepatorenal Syndrome
Ammonia buildup
Varices
Edema

Ascites
Spider veins
Clotting dysfunction
Infection, Itchy
Tired
Encephalopathy
Splenomegaly (enlarged spleen due to portal hypertension)

Patients with liver cirrhosis can develop ascites, which is fluid that builds up in the abdomen due to portal hypertension. You will often see a yellow tint in these patients (jaundice), which is caused by an increased bilirubin. When the liver can't process toxins, the ammonia level will build up also and cause encephalopathy, ranging anywhere from somnolence to coma. The liver is responsible for the synthesis of many clotting factors, so these patients will have a harder time coagulating. Hepatorenal Syndrome can eventually develop, in which a vicious cycle happens where the liver disease causes decreased renal perfusion. This eventually leads to kidney dysfunction or failure, and in turn, toxins build up in the body, worsening the liver disease. The portal hypertension can also cause an enlarged spleen, spider veins, edema, and esophageal varices. (Engorged veins in the esophagus that are more prone to bleeding). In addition, these patients often have flaky or itchy skin and are more susceptible to infection.

Hepatitis Transmission

A and E: If it's a vowel, watch the bowel (fecal, oral)
B: **B**ody Fluids (blood, semen, saliva)
C: **C**irculation, "**C**-men" (blood, semen)
D: **D**rops of Blood (blood)

Hepatitis **A** and **E** are both transmitted via the fecal oral route. So, if it's a vowel watch the bowel (GI tract). Hepatitis **B** is transmitted through **B**ody fluids, such as blood, semen, and saliva. Hepatitis **C** is transmitted though **C**irculation (blood) and **C**-men (semen). Hepatitis **D** is transmitted only through the blood (**D**rops of blood).

Kidney Disease – Symptoms

KIDNEY

K+ increased (potassium – and other electrolytes)

Increased BUN/Creatinine

Decreased GFR/Urine

Nausea

Edema

h**Y**pertension

Patients with kidney problems usually have many other problems also. Because it can't be excreted properly, the potassium level is often increased. Other electrolytes can be affected, but potassium is of the most concern. BUN and creatinine are markers for kidney function, so they should be monitored closely. They are usually elevated in kidney disease. These patients will also have a slower GFR (Glomerular Filtration Rate) and decreased urine production. Nausea is common, as is edema, due to the inability to rid the body of excess fluid. High blood pressure will eventually occur, typically because of this increased fluid in the body.

PSYCH/NEURO SYSTEM

Alzheimer's Disease – Symptoms

5 A's

Anomia (can't remember names of things)

Apraxia (using objects inappropriately)

Aphasia (unable to express feelings with voice)

Amnesia (memory loss)

Agnosia (can't recognize familiar senses, such as taste, sounds, etc)

Alzheimer's disease is progressive and degenerative form of dementia. These patients often can't remember the names of things, can't recognize familiar senses, and have a general loss of memory. They also have a difficult time using objects appropriately and have trouble expressing their feelings through their voice. These symptoms usually start out mild and may come and go. But they get worse as time goes by.

Bipolar Disorder – Depressive

DEAD SWAMP

Depressed mood
Energy loss
Anhedonia
Death thoughts (suicide)

Sleep disturbances
Worthlessness
Appetite loss
Mentation decreased
Psychomotor - agitation

Alternative...

SPACE GRADS

Sleep disturbances
Pleasure/interest (lack of)
Agitation
Concentration (lack of)
Energy (lack of)

Guilt
Retardation in movement

Appetite disturbance

Depressed mood

Suicidal thoughts

Bipolar disorder is characterized by changing periods of manic behavior and depressive behavior. In the depressive phase, these patients have suicidal thoughts, are easily agitated, and are unable to concentrate. They often lack interest in things, have feelings of guilt, and a loss of appetite. They can be slow-moving and have a lack of energy.

Bipolar Disorder – Manic Episodes

FIDGETS

Flight of ideas
Indiscretion, **I**nsomnia
Distractibility
Grandiosity
Extra activity
Talkative
Sleep deficit

Alternative...

DIG FAST

Distractibility
Indiscretion, **I**nsomnia
Grandiosity

Flight of Ideas
Activity increase
Sleep deficit
Talkative

Bipolar disorder is characterized by changing periods of manic behavior and depressive behavior. In the manic phase, these patients can't seem to sit still. They are easily distracted, very talkative, and go from idea to idea. They often have delusions of grandiosity and have trouble getting to sleep.

Cranial Nerves - Names

<u>O</u>h <u>O</u>h <u>O</u>h <u>T</u>o <u>T</u>ouch <u>A</u>nd <u>F</u>eel <u>A</u> <u>G</u>irl's <u>V</u>agina <u>A</u>nd <u>H</u>einie

I.   **O**lfactory
II.   **O**ptic
III.   **O**culomotor
IV.   **T**rochlear
V.   **T**rigeminal
VI.   **A**bducens
VII.   **F**acial
VIII.   **A**coustic (vestibulocochlear)
IX.   **G**lossopharyngeal
X.   **V**agus
XI.   **A**ccessory (spinal)
XII.   **H**ypoglossal

Cranial Nerves – Innervation

<u>S</u>ome <u>S</u>ay <u>M</u>arry <u>M</u>oney, <u>B</u>ut <u>M</u>y <u>B</u>rother <u>S</u>ays <u>B</u>ig <u>B</u>oobs <u>M</u>atter <u>M</u>ost

I.   **S**ensory
II.   **S**ensory
III.   **M**otor
IV.   **M**otor

V.   **B**oth

VI.   **M**otor

VII. **B**oth

VIII. **S**ensory

IX.   **B**oth

X.   **B**oth

XI.   **M**otor

XII. **M**otor

CVA – Symptoms

BE FAST

Balance (uncoordinated movements)
Eyes (blurry vision)

Facial Droop
Arm weakness
Speech slurred
Tachycardia

Patients who are having a stroke don't usually know what's happening to them. This is why it is so important for us to recognize the symptoms quickly. Obvious signs are slurred speech, facial droop, and weakness on one side of the body. They may also have blurred vision and a high heart rate. Because of the weakness on one side, you may also see problems with their balance.

Decorticate vs Decereberate

DecortiCate – Flexion (Arms Close)
DecerebeRate – Extension (Arms Release)

Decorticate posturing is a term to describe when a person's body stiffens with their arms bent and fists clenched. The arms are in a flexed position, so they are considered closed. Decereberate posturing is when the arms and legs are stiff, straight out, with the head arched backwards. In this case, the arms are extended, or 'released.' Both of these postures usually indicate severe damage to the brain, but decereberate is typically a more ominous sign.

Dementia – Differential Diagnosis

DEMENTIA

Drugs and Alcohol

Eyes and **E**ars

Metabolic and Endocrine disorders

Emotional disorders

Neurologic disorders

Tumors and **T**rauma

Infection

Arteriovascular disease

Dementia represents many neurological disorders that are progressive and affect ability to think and remember things. Some examples include Alzheimer's disease, vascular dementia, and Parkinson's dementia. Before you classify someone with such diseases, it's important to do a differential diagnosis to rule out other causes. Make sure it's not drugs, alcohol, infection, a tumor, trauma of some sort, or arteriovascular disease. Check for problems with vision and hearing to make sure something like that isn't making them seem demented. Some metabolic, endocrine, and other neurological disorders can also mimic dementia.

Glasgow Coma Scale (GCS)

Total score of 15 Possible (Eyes, Motor, Verbal)

Eye Opening – <u>4</u> Eyes (with glasses)
Motor – V<u>6</u> Engine
Verbal – Jackson <u>5</u>

<u>EYES</u> (4 Possible Points)

1. <u>E</u>yes are shut (no response)

2. "<u>Y</u>ikes" (eyes open to pain)

3. <u>E</u>ars (eyes open to voice)

4. <u>S</u>pontaneous eye opening

<u>Motor (**OLDBEN** – 6 Possible Points)</u>

1. <u>O</u>beys Commands

2. <u>L</u>ocalizes to pain

3. <u>D</u>raws away (withdraws from pain)

4. <u>B</u>end (flexion/decorticate response to pain)

5. <u>E</u>xtension (decereberate response to pain)

6. <u>N</u>o response

<u>Verbal (**VOWEL** - 5 Possible Points)</u>

1. <u>V</u>oiceless

2. <u>O</u>bscure (incomprehensible)

3. <u>W</u>eird words (Inappropriate words)

4. <u>E</u>rratic (confused words)

5. <u>L</u>egit (normal)

Increased Intracranial Pressure (ICP) – Symptoms

Cushing's Triad (Hypertension, Bradycardia, Irregular Respirations) is easy to remember with this mnemonic:

RIB

Respirations Irregular/Decreased
Increased BP (Hypertension)
Bradycardia

When there is too much cerebrospinal fluid in the brain and spinal cord, the intracranial pressure will increase. This can be due to various reasons, but will often cause hypertension, bradycardia, and irregular respirations. Collectively, this is known as Cushing's Triad.

Increased Intracranial Pressure (ICP) – Treatment

MOCHA MOM

Monitor ICP
Osmotic diuretics
Corticosteroids
Hyperventilate
Antipyretics

Muscle relaxants
Oxygen
Maintain CO and cerebral perfusion

When there is too much cerebrospinal fluid in the brain and spinal cord, the intracranial pressure will increase. This can be due to various reasons, but can be treated with hyperventilation, osmotic diuretics, oxygen, muscle relaxants, antipyretics, and corticosteroids. While treating, make sure you are vigilant in monitoring intracranial pressure changes. Try to maintain the cardiac output and cerebral perfusion when using these modalities.

Meningitis – Signs/Symptoms

SHIT HAPPENS

Seizures
High temp (fever)
Impaired (confused)
Tired

Headache
Altered mental status
Photophobia
Petechiae on trunk/extremities
Emesis
Neck stiffness
Sensitivity to sound

Meningitis is when the brain and spinal cord become inflamed. The culprit is usually infection, viral or bacterial. Some common symptoms include seizures, fever, confusion, tiredness, headache, photophobia (sensitivity to light), nausea, neck stiffness, sensitivity to sounds, and petechiae on the trunk and extremities. A bacterial infection is usually much worse and progresses very quickly. Antibiotics must be given in addition to supportive measures. For a viral infection, antivirals may be given, but aren't typically successful. This form of meningitis will just have to run its course while the symptoms are treated.

Maslow's Hierarchy of Needs

<u>P</u>eople <u>S</u>hould <u>L</u>ive <u>E</u>very <u>S</u>econd (Basic to higher level)

<u>S</u>elf-Actualization
<u>E</u>steem
<u>L</u>ove/belonging
<u>S</u>afety
<u>P</u>hysiological

For Maslow's Hierarchy of needs, start from the bottom (the most basic) and work your way up. In general, most of us go through life in this order, not moving on to the next level until the previous one has been realized. Physiological needs are considered the most basic, such as food, water, and shelter. Once these have been met, a person can then be compelled to seek out safety, including physical, emotional, health, and financial. Once safety is at a level a person is comfortable with, they will begin to seek out love and the feeling of belonging to a group (family, friends, co-workers). The next level is esteem, in which people aim to achieve things that bring self-esteem and esteem from others. Finally, self-actualization is at the top of the hierarchy. Usually, this can't be attained until the levels below are realized. Here, people are trying to attain something that will bring ultimate satisfaction and feeling of accomplishment. For example, a goal is achieved, a soulmate is found, happiness is obtained. This level could be anything and is really up to each individual person to decide what they are going for.

Multiple Sclerosis – Symptoms

DANISH

Dysdiadochokinesia

Ataxia

Nystagmus

Intentional tremor

Scanning speech

Hypotonia

Alternative...

UNWATCHED

Urinary retention

Nystagmus

Weakness (may progress to paralysis)

Ataxia

Tinnitus

Constipation

Hard of hearing

Eyes (blurred vision, diplopia)

Dysarthria, **D**ysphagia

Multiple Sclerosis is a disease which happens when the covers that insulate the nerve cells in the spinal cord and the brain become damaged. Because of this, it is considered a demyelinating disease. Symptoms can vary from patient to patient and depend on the progression of the disease. Some of the things you might see include urinary retention, weakness, constipation, blurred vision, and tinnitus (ringing ears). Many patients experience dysdiadochokinesia, which means they aren't able to make rapid, alternating movements. Ataxia means they don't have coordination of muscle movements. Nystagmus is involuntary eye movement. Intentional tremor is a low frequency tremor in which the person attempts to move an extremity to a certain spot, but goes slightly farther or shorter. Scanning speech refers to words that get broken up into syllables with a clear pause in many cases. Hypotonia is decreased muscle tone.

Neurogenic Shock – Causes

BAMS

Brain injury

Anesthesia (spinal)

Meds

Spinal cord injury (above T5)

In neurogenic shock, the autonomic pathways of the spinal cord are interrupted, leading to hypotension and often bradycardia. Some of the causes include brain injury, certain medications, spinal cord injuries that occur above T5, and spinal anesthesia (too much). Decreased systemic vascular resistance and loss of sympathetic tone are the result. If the problem isn't spotted and corrected quickly, then it can lead to organ damage and eventually death.

Neurogenic Shock – Symptoms

BUSHED

Bradycardia

Unopposed vagal activity

Skin warm and flushed

Hypotension

Erection (priapism – prolonged erection without arousal)

Decreased SVR

In neurogenic shock, the autonomic pathways of the spinal cord are interrupted, leading to hypotension and often bradycardia. This is caused by the decreased systemic vascular resistance and loss of sympathetic tone. If the problem isn't spotted and corrected quickly, then it can lead to organ damage and eventually death. In addition, other common symptoms include flushed skin, prolonged erection without arousal, and unopposed vagal activity (due to the loss of sympathetic tone).

Parkinson's Disease – Symptoms

SMART

Shuffling gait

Mask-like facies

Akinesia, bradykinesia

Rigidity

Tremor

Parkinson's disease is caused by a lack of dopamine that is normally produced by neurons in the brain. When these neurons become damaged, as is the case in Parkinson's, they are unable to produce the dopamine. This progressive disease causes a range of symptoms, but can eventually lead to tremor, rigidity, shuffling gait, akinesia/bradykinesia, and mask-like facies. Bradykinesia is very slow voluntary movement, while akinesia is the lack of control of voluntary movements. Mask-like facies refers to the lack of facial expression these patients often exhibit. Because they show no emotion, it often looks like a mask instead of a face.

Pupils – Exam

PERRLA

Pupils

Equal

Round and

Reactive to

Light and

Accommodation

When performing an eye exam, use PERRLA to make sure you don't forget to check something. In regard to the pupils, you want to make sure they are equal in size, round (not misshapen), and reactive to light (constrict) and accommodation. Accommodation means the pupils should constrict when focusing on a near object and dilate when focusing on an object that is farther away. They should constrict in response to light and dilate in response to darkness.

Pupils – Mydriasis (Dilation) Causes

AAA **S**outh

Antihistamines

Antidepressants

Anticholinergics (e.g. Atropine)

Sympathomimetics

Aside from naturally reacting to light and darkness, some medications can cause the pupils to dilate and constrict. Medications that can cause pupil dilation (mydriasis) include antihistamines (diphenhydramine), antidepressants (amitriptyline), anticholinergics (atropine), and sympathomimetics (pseudoephedrine). Other culprits include some anti-seizure medications, Botox, Parkinson's medications, and anti-nausea medications.

Pupils – Miosis (Constriction) Causes

COMPLAINS

Clonidine

Opiates

Mushrooms/**M**uscarinic agents

Phenothiazines

Lomotil

Asleep

Insecticides

Narcotics

Stroke, **S**edatives

Aside from naturally reacting to light and darkness, some outside influences can cause the pupils to dilate and constrict. Some things that can cause pupil constriction (miosis) include clonidine, opiates, mushrooms, phenothiazines (Compazine), Lomotil, insecticides, narcotics, stroke, sedatives, and the simple act of being asleep.

Schizophrenia – Symptoms

The **CRAP** rolls **DOWNHILL**

Changes in personality
Religiosity
Autism
Peculiar behavior

Delusions
Often disorganized
Withdrawn
Negativism
Hallucinations/**H**ypersensitivity to sound, sight, and smell
Indifferent
Loss of ego
Lack of social awareness

Schizophrenia is a disease in which people see reality differently. This condition is characterized by changes in personality, peculiar behavior, delusions, hallucinations, and lack of social awareness. They often have strong feelings toward religion and they can be disorganized. They are usually withdrawn, have a negative outlook, loss of ego, and are hypersensitive to certain senses. There is sometimes a correlation with some forms of autism and schizophrenia.

Suicide Precautions

NO COMBS

NO:

COrds (phone, curtains, etc)
Matches or cigarettes
Belts
Sharps/razors

Patients who have threatened or attempted suicide should be placed on proper suicide precautions. This means leaving them alone as little as possible and making sure they don't have access to anything that can be used to harm themselves. There shouldn't be any cords, belts, curtains, or anything else that can be used in the same manner. Take away lighters and matches and make sure there aren't any sharp objects, such as razors, needles, pens/pencils, etc.

PULMONARY SYSTEM

Adventitious Lung Sounds - Crackles

CRACKLES

Crepitations

Rales

Atelectasis

Collapsed Alveoli

Krispy (sounds like Rice Krispies)

Lower Lobes

Edema

Shortness of Breath

Crackles are caused by collapsed or fluid-filled alveoli. This can sometimes be caused by pneumonia from a bad cold or flu. It may also happen after surgery when the patient is not taking deep enough breaths. It most often effects the lower lobes of the lungs and sounds like Rice Krispies popping. Rales is another term for crackles.

Adventitious Lung Sounds – Ronchi

RHONCHI

Rattling

Heavy sleep (snoring sound)

Obstruction of fluid

Narrowing

Coarse

Heard more in larger airways

Inspiration or Expiration

Rhonchi is usually heard when there is thick mucus present, like with a bad cold or pneumonia. It is a rattling sound that resembles snoring. It can be heard when the patient is breathing in or out, and usually can be heard over larger airways. Typically, rhonchi can be cleared with coughing. Get that patient some mucinex!

Adventitious Lung Sounds – Stridor

STRIDOR

Sounds harsh, high pitched

Turbulent air flow

Racemic Epinephrine

Intubate?

Decadron (steroids)

Obstructed airway

Raise head of bed

Stridor happens when something is impeding airflow into or out of the lungs. Examples of this include epiglottitis, tumor, or foreign body. It is also common in children with croup. It sounds high pitched and harsh due to the turbulent airflow. You can try treating with steroids, such as Decadron or a bronchodilator, such as epinephrine. Raising the head of the bed may also help to decrease the effect of the obstruction. Intubation is always a possibility and is something that may be needed if other treatment options fail.

Adventitious Lung Sounds – Wheeze

WHEEZE

Whistling

High Pitched

Emphysema, asthma, COPD

Expiratory wheeze more common

Zyrtec (allergies common)

Epinephrine (or other beta-agonists, e.g. Albuterol)

This is a sound due to narrowing of the airways, most commonly heard upon expiration. These patients may have allergies, asthma, COPD, or emphysema. It sounds like a high-pitched whistling sound as they struggle to get air out. Prompt treatment with a beta-agonist, such as albuterol or epinephrine, is a must.

Alkalosis vs Acidosis

ROME

Respiratory – **O**pposite
Metabolic – **E**qual

If the alkalosis is due to a Respiratory cause, pH will be high and pCO2 will be low
If the acidosis is due to a Respiratory cause, pH will be low and pCO2 will be high

If the alkalosis is due to a Metabolic cause, pH and HCO3 will be high
If the acidosis is due to a Metabolic cause, pH and HCO3 will be low

Learning how to do abgs can be a pain in the butt. This should help you remember, but you're still going to have to learn the basics first.

Step 1:
Look at the pH (Is it high, low, or normal?)
High (> 7.45) = Alkalosis
Low (< 7.35) = Acidosis
Normal (7.35 – 7.45)

If it's normal, then you're good and don't need to do anything else (In most cases). If it's high or low, then we need to find out why.

Step 2:
Look at the PaCO2 (Is it high, low, or normal?)

High CO2 (>45) with low pH = Respiratory Acidosis
Low CO2 (<35) with high pH = Respiratory Alkalosis

If it's neither of these, then let's go on to HCO3. It could be a metabolic problem.

Step 3:
Look at the HCO3 (Is it high, low, or normal?)
High HCO3 (>26) with high pH = Metabolic Alkalosis
Low HCO3 (<22) with low pH = Metabolic Acidosis

Step 4:
Determine if the acidosis or alkalosis is fully compensated, partially compensated, or uncompensated. This is a little more advanced and is something we tackle more in depth in other publications and on our web site.

Asthma – Symptoms

COW BASH

Coughing

Obstruction

Wheezing

Bronchospasm

Avoid Irritants

Shortness of breath

Hard to get air out

Asthma is a disease of the lungs characterized by inflammation and narrowing of the airways. It is basically an overreaction by the body. It often causes coughing and wheezing due to the obstruction. The irritated airways can lead to bronchospasm and shortness of breath. Any irritants, such as allergies, smoke, and sprays should be avoided.

Asthma – Treatment

ASTHMA

Adrenergics (B2 agonists – e.g. Albuterol)
Steroids
Theophylline
Hydration
Mask (oxygen)
Antibiotics, **A**nticholinergics

Asthma is a disease of the lungs characterized by inflammation and narrowing of the airways. It is basically an overreaction of the body. They are different treatments for active asthma attacks and maintenance/prevention of an attack. This mnemonic is easy to remember because it is the word, "asthma." First treatment is usually adrenergics, such as albuterol. Steroids are often reserved for maintenance or briefly after an attack is under control. Sometimes theophylline is used, which relaxes the smooth muscle of the airway and decreases the response to stimuli. Fluids, oxygen, anticholinergics, and antibiotics (if infection is the suspected cause) may also be ordered.

COPD – Symptoms

CRAP WIPE

Chronic cough/**C**lubbing of fingers
Round barrel chest
Accessory muscle use
Prolonged expiratory time

Wheezing
Increased work of breathing
Purse-lip breathing
Easily fatigued

Chronic Obstructive Pulmonary Disease (COPD) is usually caused by long-term cigarette smoking, but can also be from exposure to irritants, and a small number from genetic deficiencies. These patients have difficulty getting air out of their lungs, which also makes it difficult to get air back in. This progressive disease will eventually lead to a chronic cough, clubbing of the fingers (distorted angle of nail bed), wheezing, prolonged expiratory time, accessory muscle use, and increased work of breathing. In an attempt to get air in, they purse their lips and are easily fatigued. Eventually COPD patients may develop a barrel chest, in which it bulges out in a round shape that looks a barrel. This happens because the lungs are chronically overinflated due to the inability to get air out. This constant inflation slowly spreads the ribcage to make it have this appearance. The term COPD also represents emphysema, chronic bronchitis, and refractory asthma.

COPD – Treatment

ABCDEF

Aminophylline
Bronchodilators
Chest physiotherapy
Deliver oxygen
Expectorant
Force fluids

Chronic Obstructive Pulmonary Disease (COPD) is usually caused by long-term cigarette smoking, but can also be from exposure to irritants, and a small number from genetic deficiencies. These patients have difficulty getting air out of their lungs, which also makes it difficult to get air back in. Treatment might include supplemental oxygen, bronchodilators, fluids, aminophylline, expectorant (such as guaifenesin), and chest physiotherapy (percussion, vibration, etc). The term COPD also represents emphysema, chronic bronchitis, and refractory asthma.

Lungs – Lobes

How many lobes does each lung have?

Right Lung – 3 Lobes
Left Lung – 2 Lobes

Imagine a big **R**. It takes **3** separate lines to create this letter (the straight vertical line, the little loop, and the slanted line down).

Imagine a big **L**. It takes **2** separate lines to create this letter (The straight vertical line and the straight horizontal line).

When you're first starting out in nursing school, you may have trouble remembering which side of the lungs has two or three lobes. The left has 2 lobes (upper and lower) while the right has 3 lobes (upper, middle, and lower). Follow this mnemonic to help you remember whenever you're having a brain fart.

Pulmonary Edema – Treatment

MAD DOG

Morphine
Aminophylline
Digitalis

Diuretics
Oxygen
Gases (ABGs)

Pulmonary edema is a problem in which too much fluid gets in the lungs. Treatment includes morphine to help with anxiety and preload reduction, along with aminophylline to dilate the airway. Digitalis can be used to increase the calcium in the heart, thereby strengthening the contraction it provides. Stronger contraction means better blood flow and clearing of fluid that has backed up. Oxygen may be used, as well as diuretics to reduce the amount of fluid. Regular arterial blood gases should be obtained to evaluate treatment and progression.

Pulmonary Embolism (PE) – Symptoms

CATFISH

Chest pain, **C**ough

Arrest (cardiac arrest)

Tachycardia

Fever

Increased anxiety

Shortness of breath

Hypotension

A pulmonary embolism happens when a blood clot breaks free and gets lodged in one of the arteries that lead to the lungs. Common symptoms include chest pain, cough, tachycardia, fever, anxiety, shortness of breath, and hypotension. If the clot is big enough and is not treated quickly, cardiac arrest will be imminent. Pulmonary embolisms are very dangerous and could lead to death very quickly, even in seemingly young and healthy patients.

Pulmonary Embolism (PE) – Treatment

FATS

Filter (IVC filter)
Anticoagulants
Thrombolytics
Symptoms (Treat symptoms – oxygen, pain meds, CPR, vent)

A pulmonary embolism happens when a blood clot breaks free and gets lodged in one of the arteries that lead to the lungs. Initial treatment will include responding to the symptoms. These patients will need to be stabilized before doing anything else. Once stable, thrombolytics may be ordered to help dissolve the clot. Anticoagulants can be given to thin the blood to prevent future clots. An IVC filter can also be placed to help stop any future dislodged clots from traveling any further than the filter itself.

Tuberculosis – Medications

PRIEST

Pyrazinamide
Rifampin
Isoniazid
Ethambutol
Streptomycin

Tuberculosis is an infection that can affect any part of the body, but most often occurs in the lungs. It is caused by bacteria called Mycobacterium tuberculosis. These treatments are difficult to remember due to the complexity of the drugs names, but hopefully this mnemonic will help some. Common medications used to treat tuberculosis include pyrazinamide, rifampin, isoniazid, ethambutol, and streptomycin.

Tuberculosis – Symptoms

WATCH for these:

Weakness
Anorexia
Temperature (fever, night sweats)
Chronic cough, **C**hest pain
Hemoptysis

Tuberculosis is an infection that can affect any part of the body, but most often occurs in the lungs. It is caused by bacteria called Mycobacterium tuberculosis. Common symptoms include generalized weakness and fatigue, loss of appetite, fever, night sweats, chronic cough, and chest pain. The cough is often accompanied by blood-tinged sputum (hemoptysis).

OB/
PEDIATRICS

Evaluation of Episiotomy Healing

DARED

Discharge
Approximation
Redness
Edema, **E**cchymosis
Drainage

Alternative...

DREAD

Discharge
Redness
Edema, **E**cchymosis
Approximation
Drainage

An episiotomy is a cut that the doctor makes during childbirth at the base of the vagina. This is done during deliveries that are difficult in an effort to prevent rupture as the baby comes out. Once delivered, the incision is stitched back up and must be kept clean in the days to follow to prevent infection.

Fetal Accelerations/Decelerations

VEAL CHOP

Variable Decelerations – **C**ord Compression
Early Decelerations – **H**ead Compression
Accelerations – **O**kay!
Late Decelerations – **P**lacental Insufficiency

Alternative...

Very **D**irty **C**hildren
Variable **D**ecelerations – **C**ord Compression

Every **D**ay **H**ero
Early **D**ecelerations – **H**ead Compression

Lucky **D**og **P**aws
Late **D**ecelerations – **P**lacental Insufficiency

VEAL CHOP is the most popular one and probably the easiest to remember. But if you wanted something a little quirkier, use the alternative. A deceleration is when the fetal heart rate goes below the baseline. Acceleration, therefore, means that the fetal heart rate increases above the baseline. Early deceleration happens slightly before or with a contraction, recovering to baseline by the time it's over. This would indicate that the baby's head is being compressed during contraction. Late deceleration doesn't recover to baseline until after the contraction is over. This usually means that there is insufficient perfusion to the placenta. Variable decelerations mean that the drop in fetal heart rate could come before, during, or after a contraction. This usually means the umbilical cord is being compressed. Accelerations are usually not a sign of any major underlying problem.

Fetal Non-Stress Test

<u>Non</u>-reactive

<u>Non</u>-stress test

is

<u>Not</u> good!

One of the tests to determine fetal well-being is the non-stress test. In this test, the baby's heart rate is monitored to see if it accelerates during movement. It is a good sign if the baby's heart rate speeds up during movement. This would be considered a "reactive" result. If there is little to no acceleration during movement, then it would be considered a "non-reactive" result. This can sometimes be an ominous sign.

Fetal Well-Being Tests

ALONE

Amniocentesis

L/S Ratio

Oxytocin test

Non-stress test

Estriol levels

Alternative...

LOANED

L/S ratio

Oxytocin Test

Amniocentesis

Non-stress test

Estriol levels

Doppler ultrasound

An important part of pregnancy is making sure the baby is doing well through various means. This is not an exhaustive list, but is good to get the basics down. An amniocentesis is where a needle is inserted into the uterus to get a sample of amniotic fluid that can be tested against many possible abnormalities. The L/S ratio stands for lecithin-sphingomyelin, a test that determines how mature the fetal lung development is. The oxytocin challenge test is also known as the contraction stress test.

This is usually done around 34 weeks along in the pregnancy and assesses how the fetus will manage contractions of childbirth. The non-stress test monitors the baby's heartbeat and movement. If the non-stress test is "reactive," it tells us that the baby's heartbeat rises with movement. If it is "non-reactive," it tells us that the heartbeat doesn't rise with movement. It's a better sign to have a "reactive" non-stress test. Estriol levels can be measured from samples of urine or blood from the mother. The results can tell of possible chromosomal abnormalities and other potential issues. The doppler ultrasound is what every pregnant woman gets if she is seeing an obstetrician throughout her pregnancy. This can show physical characteristics of the baby, and can help in determining things like size, weight, and sex.

Postpartum Assessment

Humble

Homan's Sign

Uterus

Movement of bowels

Breast, **B**ladder

Lochia

Episiotomy, **E**motional status

Alternative...

BUMBLE BEE

Breasts

Uterus

Maintain comfort

Bowel function

Lochia

Episiotomy healing

Bladder function

Emotional status

Evaluate for DVT (Homan's Sign)

During a postpartum assessment, both breasts should be palpated, checking for engorgement. Check the nipples for sores and document their appearance. The uterus (fundus) should be checked and the height, position, and tone should be recorded. Check for bowel sounds, give stool softeners, and feel for distention. Record urine volumes and appearance, and check for bladder distention if not voiding. Watch for signs of urinary tract infection. Assess for appearance, amount, and odor. Excessive bleeding should be reported to the doctor. If an episiotomy was done, check for redness, edema, ecchymosis, discharge, and approximation (REEDA). Homan's Sign is when there is discomfort or pain behind the knee when you dorsiflex the foot. This could indicate the presence of DVT. Check the mother's emotional status to make sure she is handling things appropriately. Offer emotional support as needed.

Pre-eclampsia – Medications

My **L**oving **B**aby **H**as **D**emands

Magnesium

Labetalol

Betamethasone

Hydralazine

Dexamethasone

Pre-eclampsia is a problem that can happen during pregnancy, in which hypertension is accompanied by large amounts of protein in the urine. It usually happens after the 20th week. If seizures happen, then it is termed 'eclampsia.' To prevent this, magnesium is given to raise the seizure threshold. Labetalol and hydralazine may be given to treat the high blood pressure. Steroids, such as betamethasone and dexamethasone can be given to help develop the baby's lungs as much as possible in case early delivery is necessary.

Severe Pre-Eclampsia - Symptoms

HELLP

Hemolysis
Elevated **L**iver enzymes
Low **P**latelet count

Alternative...

TRIPLE

Thrombocytopenia
Renal Insufficiency
Intracranial disturbance
Proteinuria, **P**ressure (BP) is high
LFT Elevation
Edema

When does Pre-eclampsia become Eclampsia?
Here's a rhyme to help you remember:

If the patient has seizures and you agree
It's now Eclampsia (drop the "pre")

INHERITED

DISORDERS

Congenital Cyanotic Heart Defects

One big **trunk** (**Trunc**us Arteriosus)
Two interchanged vessels (Transposition of the Great Vessels)
Three: **Tri**cuspid Atresia
Four: **Tetra**logy of Fallot
Five words: Total Anomalous Pulmonary Venous Return

Alternative...

5 T's

Truncus Arteriosus
Transposition of the Great Vessels
Tricuspid Atresia
Tetralogy of Fallot
Total Anomalous Pulmonary Venous Return

Cystic Fibrosis – Features

ABCDEFGHI

Autosomal recessive

Bronchiectasis

Chloride channel block, **C**iliary dysfunction

Diabetes

Exocrine pancreatic failure

Fat malabsorption

Gall stones, **G**ene mutation on chromosome 7

Hepatic cirrhosis, **H**emoptysis

Infertility

Just follow the alphabet for this mnemonic. Cystic fibrosis is an autosomal recessive disease, meaning that one abnormal gene was obtained from each parent. Bronchiectasis is a common feature in these patients, so they have lots of mucus in the airway that is difficult to clear out. The Cystic Fibrosis transmembrane conductance regulator is a protein and calcium channel which is blocked in the disease. This causes an inability to regulate the epithelial fluid transportation in the lungs and pancreas, among others. Inadequate mucociliary clearance plays a role in cystic fibrosis, but don't confuse this disease with ciliary dyskinesia. The increased mucus can damage the pancreas, leading to diabetes and exocrine pancreatic failure. Fat isn't absorbed as well, and these patients often present with gallstones. Cystic fibrosis can also cause liver cirrhosis, infertility, and hemoptysis (coughing up blood-tinged sputum).

Cystic Fibrosis – Treatment

B DAMP

Breathing exercises, **B**ronchodilators
Diet (increase protein)
Aerosol therapy, **A**ntibiotics
Mucolytics
Postural drainage, **P**ancreatic enzymes

Cystic fibrosis doesn't have a cure, so we just have to treat the symptoms the best we can. This can include breathing exercises and bronchodilators, increased protein in the diet, antibiotics, aerosol therapy, mucolytics, postural drainage, and pancreatic enzymes. In some cases, a lung transplant may be done.

Hemophilia – Differentiating between A, B, and C

Hemophilia A: Factor VIII Deficiency
A̲: **A̲te** (8)

Hemophilia B: Factor IX Deficiency (Christmas Disease)
B̲: I **B̲**elieved in **S̲anta** at **9̲** years old (9)

Hemophilia C: Factor XI Deficiency
C̲: **C̲a**l**l** me (11)

Hemophilia A is a deficiency of coagulation factor VIII (8). Hemophilia B is a deficiency of coagulation factor IX (9) and is also known as Christmas Disease. Hemophilia C is a deficiency of factor XI (11). This mnemonic can be useful when trying to remember how to differentiate between the three.

Sickle Cell Crisis - Symptoms

SICKLE

Stroke risk

Infection

Cell clumping

Killer pain

Leg ulcers

Enlarged spleen

Sickle Cell Disease is when atypical hemoglobin molecules (Hemoglobin S) are present in the bloodstream. This distorts the red blood cells so that they appear crescent in shape (sickle). Common symptoms in a sickle cell crisis include severe pain, infection, leg ulcers, and enlarged spleen. These patients are at an increased risk of stroke and other thromboembolic events.

Sickle Cell Crisis – Treatment

MOTH

Meds for pain
Oxygen
Transfusions
Hydration

Sickle Cell Disease is when atypical hemoglobin molecules (Hemoglobin S) are present in the bloodstream. This distorts the red blood cells so that they appear crescent in shape (sickle). Treatment for this disease may include oxygen, blood transfusions, and hydration. Pain medication will be necessary due to the extreme pain that a sickle cell crisis causes.

MISC.
MNEMONICS

Anaphylactic Shock – Common Causes

Foot In Mouth

Food allergies (peanuts, seafood, eggs)
Insect stings (bees, wasps, ants)
Medication reaction

Anaphylactic shock happens when there is an overreaction of the body's defense mechanisms to an offending substance. It is usually very rapidly progressing and could lead to death if not treated quickly. Common causes include allergies (food or otherwise), stings from insects (such as bees, wasps, and ants), and reaction to medications.

Anaphylactic Shock – Symptoms

STARFISH

Swelling
Tachycardia
Arrest
Rapid onset
Flushing
Itching
Shortness of Breath (bronchospasm, laryngeal edema)
Hypotension

Anaphylactic shock happens when there is an overreaction of the body's defense mechanisms to an offending substance. It is usually very rapidly progressing and could lead to death if not treated quickly. Common symptoms include swelling, tachycardia, respiratory and cardiac arrest, flushing skin, itching, shortness of breath, and hypotension. Once the airway is affected, the swelling could cause the mouth and throat to close up, so these patients have to be taken care of without delay.

Antidotes

Coumadin – Vitamin K
Cold Vampire

Heparin – Protamine Sulfate
Hot Priest

Benzodiazepines – Romazicon (Flumazenil)
Banana Republic

Opiates – Naloxone (Narcan)
Old Navy

Tylenol – Mucomyst
Time Magazine

Beta Blockers – Glucagon
Bradycardia's Gone

Aphasia vs Aphagia vs Dysphasia vs Dysphagia

Aphasia: Speech (unable to speak)
Dysphasia: Speech (difficulty expressing through speaking)
Aphagia: Swallowing (unable to swallow)
Dysphagia: Swallowing (difficulty swallowing)

If it ends in **Sia**, it has to do with **S**peech

If it ends in **Gia**, it has to do with **GI** (swallowing)

If it starts with **A**, there is **A**bsence (Inability to speak or swallow)

If it starts with **D**, there is **D**ifficulty (Difficulty with speaking or swallowing)

Keep in mind that a lot of people use these terms interchangeably. Be sure to see if the term given matches their symptoms.

Breast Assessment

MELON

Mammary Changes
Examine patient history
Lumps
Other symptoms
Nipple changes

When doing a breast assessment, always remember to be discrete and respectful. Look for any apparent changes that may deviate from the norm. Examine the patient's history and look for lumps, deformities, changes in the nipples, or any other symptoms that may have been reported. Remind the patient to do self-breast exams at home.

Cancer Warning Signs

BE CAUTIOUS

Bleeding or discharge (that isn't normal)
Extreme fatigue

Change in bowel or bladder habits
A sore that won't heal
Unexplained weight loss
Thickening of lump in breast or elsewhere
Irritating cough or hoarseness
Obvious changes in wart or mole
Unexplained anemia
Swallowing difficulty or indigestion

Cancer sucks. The earlier you can catch it, usually the better off you are. Some signs and symptoms to look out for include any bleeding or discharge that isn't normal, extreme fatigue, change in bowel or bladder habits, unexplained weight loss, and sores that won't heal. Other things to watch for are swallowing difficulty, unexplained anemia, persistent cough, or lumps in the breasts and other areas.

Chemotherapy Side Effects

BARFS

Bone marrow depression

Alopecia

Retching (nausea)

Fear and anxiety

Stomatitis

Patients who have cancer may sometimes have the option to receive chemotherapy. The side effects are usually awful for most people, and include severe nausea and vomiting, hair loss, and stomatitis (inflammation in the mouth and lip area). They often develop bone marrow depression, which can lead to anemia and open the patient up to infection. For obvious reasons, fear and anxiety is very common.

Compartment Syndrome – Signs/Symptoms

5 P's

Pain

Pallor

Pulse decreased/absent

Pressure increased

Paresthesia

Compartment syndrome happens when there is too much built-up pressure inside of a part of the body, which leads to lack of blood flow in that area. It most often happens in the extremities after a patient suffers a broken bone. Common symptoms include pain, pallor (paleness), decreased pulse in that area, increased pressure in that area, and paresthesia (abnormal sensation in that area).

Emergency Medications

Drugs to **LEAN** on

Lidocaine

Epinephrine

Atropine

Narcan

Alternative...

LAND A SAVE

Lidocaine

Amiodarone

Narcan

Dopamine, **D**extrose

Adenosine

Sodium Bicarbonate

Atropine

Vasopressin

Epinephrine

LEAN is good if you want something quick and basic. But I prefer LAND A SAVE, which is something you can easily do if you remember your emergency protocols. Knowing these medications will help.

Epiglottitis – Symptoms

AIR RAID

Airway closed
Increased pulse
Restlessness

Retractions
Anxiety
Inspiratory stridor
Drooling

Epiglottitis is considered a medical emergency which requires intervention before the airway is lost. It is caused by infection and causes swelling of the epiglottis. These patients often present with drooling, retractions while breathing, anxiety, inspiratory stridor, restlessness, and tachycardia. A common telltale sign is drooling while leaning forward in an effort to get more air into the lungs.

Epiglottitis – Treatment

NO FAITH

NPO
Oxygen

Fluids
Avoid examination of throat
Intubate
Tracheostomy
Humidification (cool mist)

Epiglottitis is considered a medical emergency which requires intervention before the airway is lost. It is caused by infection and causes swelling of the epiglottis. Treatments includes oxygen, fluids, and cool mist humidification. Keep these patients NPO in case surgery is needed. You will also want to avoid anything that might irritate the epiglottis, causing more swelling. This is another reason to keep food away. You should also avoid examining the throat for the same reason. If necessary, these patients may need to be intubated. If it is severe enough and a breathing tube can't be passed, then a tracheostomy may be needed.

Eyes – Abbreviations

OU, OD, OS

Both eyes are a c**OU**ple
You won't **OD** with the **Right** one
The only one **Left** is **OS**

OU – Both Eyes
OD – Right
OS – Left

This mnemonic should help you remember the medical abbreviations for right, left, and both eyes. If you are documenting both eyes, it's OU (you have a cOUple of eyes). For just the right eye, it's OD (the Right dose won't cause an overdose/OD). The left side is OS and happens to be the only one left. If you know what both eyes are and what the right eye is, then you'll know what the left eye is by process of elimination.

Lupus – Symptoms

PARANOID MD'S

Photosensitivity

Arthritis

Renal (proteinuria)

ANA Positive (Antinuclear Antibody)

Neurologic (e.g. seizure)

Oral ulcers

Immunologic (DS DNA, etc.)

Decreased blood levels (anemia, leukopenia, thrombocytopenia)

Malar rash

Discoid rash

Serositis (pleuritic, pericarditis)

Lupus is an autoimmune disease that causes widespread inflammation. Its longer name is systemic lupus erythematosus (SLE). Some common symptoms include photosensitivity, arthritis, proteinuria, ulcers in the mouth, and rashes. Watch out for anemia, leukopenia (low white blood cell count), and thrombocytopenia (low platelets). You may see some neurological manifestations, such as seizures, headaches, and sensitivity to light. Another big problem with these patients is the possibility of pleuritis and pericarditis.

Mole Assessment

ABCDE

Asymmetry

Border

Color

Diameter

Evolving

When evaluating patients for moles to determine if they are worrisome, follow this simple mnemonic. Moles that are asymmetric, have irregular edges, and a large diameter are all red flags. Moles should be close to the same color all over and not have areas of patchiness. Moles are also a cause for concern if they are evolving, meaning they have changed over time. Typical, run-of-the-mill moles will stay the same over long periods of time.

Order of Lab Draws

Stop **L**ight **R**ed **S**tay **P**ut, **G**reen **L**ight **G**o

Sterile

Light Blue

Red

SST

PST

Green

Lavender

Gray

In order to prevent cross-contamination of the additives in each tube, lab draws must done in a specific order. This mnemonic should help you remember. When the stop light is red, stay put. Green Light? Go! Start with anything that must be collected sterile. Then move on to the light blue tube, followed by red, sst (serum separating tube), pst (plasma separation tube), green, lavender, and finally gray. Keep in mind that some of these colors might possibly be different in the various sites you work in. Always follow the policies at your facility.

Sepsis – Symptoms

SEPSIS

Shivering (fever)

Extreme pain or discomfort

Pale

Shortness of breath

Ideas of death (thoughts of impending doom)

Sleepy, lethargic

Sepsis is an infection that has spread and gotten into the bloodstream. This is a life-threatening problem and can quickly lead to death if not dealt with quickly. Common symptoms include fever, pain, discomfort, shortness of breath, lethargy, paleness, and thoughts of impending doom.

Sepsis – Treatment

SHOP

Start antibiotics

Hydrate

Oxygen (support with vent if needed)

Pressors (correct hypotension)

Sepsis is an infection that has spread and gotten into the bloodstream. This is a life-threatening problem and can quickly lead to death if not dealt with quickly. Treatment includes antibiotics to treat the infection, hydration, oxygen, and vasopressors to treat hypotension. Aside from this, treating the symptoms and making the patient more comfortable would also be included in the plan.

Sprains and Strains – Treatment

RICE

Rest
Ice
Compression
Elevation

A strain happens when muscles are overstretched and the fibers tear. A sprain happens a ligament is stretched too far (it may tear or just overstretch). Patients who come in with a sprain or strain just need to follow a few simple rules to get back on their feet. The biggest thing they can do is rest the affected body part and give it time to heal. The injury should be elevated, iced, and compressed as much as possible.

Trauma Assessment

ABCDEFGHI

Airway

Breathing

Circulation

Disability

Examine

Fever (check temp)

Get vital signs

Head-to-toe assessment

Intervention

Alternative...

PLASTICS

Punctures

Lacerations

Abrasions

Swelling

Tenderness

Irregularities (deformities, discolorations)

Contusions

Scald (burns)

Wound Infection – Signs/Symptoms

SHARP

Swelling

Heat/**H**igh temp (fever)

Awful smell

Redness/**R**ed streaks

Pain/**P**urulent drainage (Pus formation)

When a wound becomes infected, there are commonly some telltale signs to warn us. There is usually swelling in the affected area and it can have an odor to it. It will probably be warm to the touch, red and irritated, and cause pain upon palpation. These patients will often have a fever and purulent drainage may be coming from the site.

That's it for now! I hope you were able to get something useful out of this book. These mnemonics helped me a lot while I was going through nursing school. When you encounter a difficult subject that you find hard to remember, try to make up some of your own. Good luck in your nursing career!

Remember to check out the web site for more books, helpful information from the blog, and nursing in general. We are constantly adding new things every day.

www.kickassnursing.com

Made in the USA
Coppell, TX
12 May 2020

25302720R00095